The Magic of Indian Ginseng – Ashwagandha

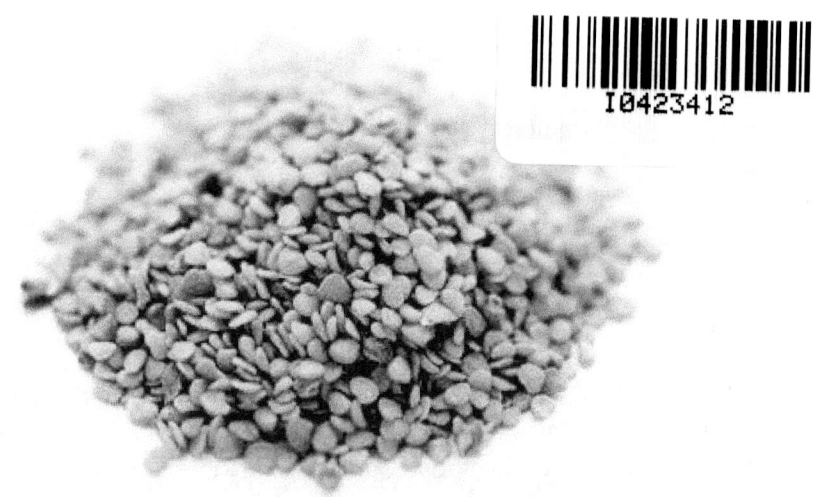

I0423412

Dueep Jyot Singh

Healthy Learning Series

Mendon Cottage Books

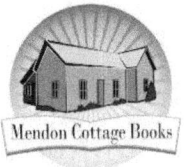

JD-Biz Publishing

Download Free Books!

http://MendonCottageBooks.com

All Rights Reserved.

No part of this publication may be reproduced in any form or by any means, including scanning, photocopying, or otherwise without prior written permission from JD-Biz Corp Copyright © 2016

All Images Licensed by Fotolia and 123RF.

Disclaimer

The information is this book is provided for informational purposes only. The information is believed to be accurate as presented based on research by the author.

The author or publisher is not responsible for the use or safety of any procedure or treatment mentioned in this book. The author or publisher is not responsible for errors or omissions that may exist.

Our books are available at

1. Amazon.com
2. Barnes and Noble
3. Itunes
4. Kobo
5. Smashwords
6. Google Play Books

Download Free Books!

http://MendonCottageBooks.com

Table of Contents

Introduction

It is amazing the amount of plants, you can see all around you, without knowing their names, or their uses, and then around 40 years later, you say, hey, I know that plant, I recognize it, it used to grow and flourish in the wild forest regions, where I spent my childhood and youth!

Well, this particular enlightenment occurred, when I saw dried plants of Withania Somnifora being uprooted by a herbalist friend, because she intended to make some herbal decoctions, concoctions, tinctures, and rejuvenating potions for friends, relatives and members of the family.

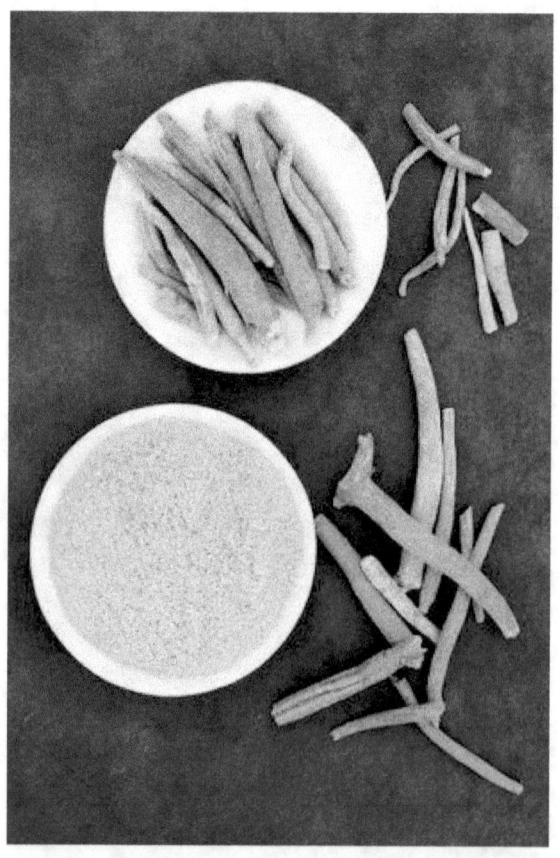

Even then, the name did not click, even though I thought I knew these red berries. We were expressly forbidden to eat them as children, so I considered them to be poisonous. So naturally, I ignored this plant as not worthy of my attention as a child.

I did not know that as an adult, this plant would be world famous all over the world as one of the most powerful sources of natural revitalizing ingredients, especially when one felt his potency, vitality, and virile strength flagging.

This plant is known as Ashwagandha for millenniums, and now more and more people in the West have found that this is an excellent, healthy, and healing source, along with Bacopa, of which I will write soon – and Emblica - which you can find here: **http://tinyurl.com/zofm2uk** – and it is no wonder that there are 7 American companies and 4 Japanese companies, which are trying to take out patents on their own products in which they have added a little bit of Ashwagandha and a little bit of ginseng!

But, as this is a natural traditional medicine used in Chinese, and alternative Indian medicine for millenniums, I do not think that any recipe with a number of ingredients picked up without bothering about the quantity and which they could have made up in the form of any jazzy modern medicine, calling it a 21st-century creation with a patent stuck onto it, could be considered to be beneficial or even healthy!

How I Got to Know about Ashwagandha

Incidentally, how I began thinking about this particular Herb, when a friend of mine sent me a message that she wanted to put this particular Indian product "ass wer gender" on her site – *grow healthy naturally* – and could I advise her on it?

I told her to write down the word and send it to me on email, because I could not make out the pronunciation- *uhhh -ash waa gain dhay, ashwayg gand haa-* and whichever way, Astrid could manage to pronounce this word, when I asked for bewildered vocal repeats.

I had not heard of this herb at all. And she called it an Indian herb? What was the scientific name? "*Why thaa naaya some e nai forra*?" Says Astrid tranquilly.

Could you be speaking of "*wee thaa niya som nee fora*?" I asked timidly.

"Is that how you pronounce it?" She said a trifle irritated. "Man, you botanists really know how to trouble us ordinary human beings with your silly pronunciations."

A bulb lit up in my brain. Were you talking about "*Ash waa gun dhaa.*"

"What?" said Astrid, and then after a bewildered moment, "whatever."

So I just requested of her that if she was talking about *Withania somnifora* also known the world over as Ashwagandha, she needed to put this healing herb on to her website and as soon as possible.

So this book is going to tell you all about the power of this particular healing herb, how you can grow it at home, how you can use its roots, and its berries to heal yourself. Also, you are going to get more information about how in company knowledge or just taking the word of others, who know not what they speak, even though they have a large number of professional alphabets behind their names, can be potentially harmful.

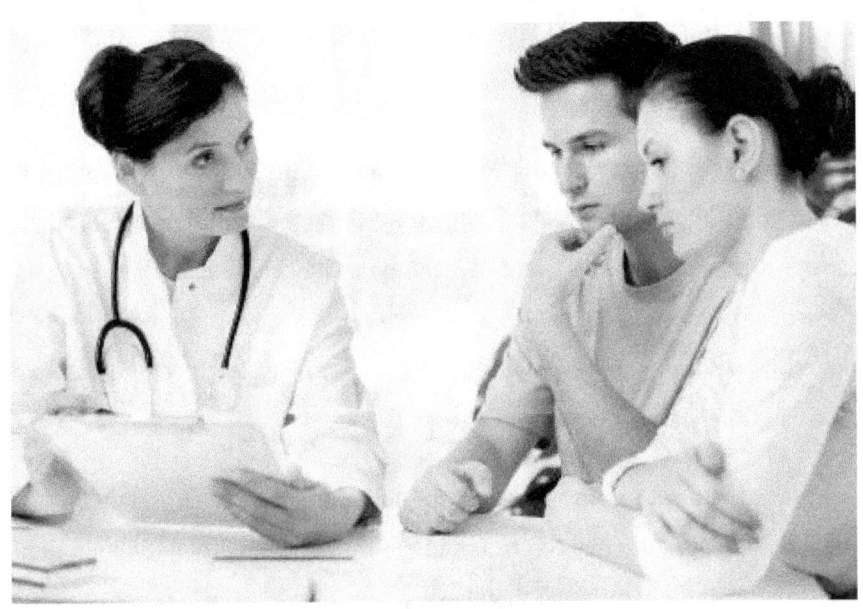

You are taking alternative medicines? You are taking herbal remedies? Don't you know that nobody has spent billions of dollars in researching the medicines that you are taking to cure yourself? It has not been proven by our doctors that you can use these herbs to cure yourself of bronchitis, asthma, or nervous strain and stress. So you had better continue taking the medicines, which I have been prescribing for you, and that reminds me, you have your last bill to pay, $2,000. Please clear that payment right now.

Is this what you are going through, when you go to a hospital?

This is the reason why so many people have started getting afraid of taking alternative medicine remedies, which could have cured them of all their ills. That is because they have been frightened by the researchers of their countries, who say that such and such medicine is going to have such and such bad side effect, when taken, and it has not been scientifically proven that that particular medicine is useful for treating one particular ailment or illness.

That is because these researchers do not know all about the correct usage or the dosage of the medicine. Also, they may be spending millions of dollars, researching on parts of the plant, which do not have any medicinal properties! This is almost as bad as a person throwing away potato tubers and telling a simple farmer, that the potato plant is useless because the leaves and the flowers were useless to eat!

So what is the use of doing research on the leaves of the Ashwagandha, when in ancient medicine, the fruit and the roots were used? And then they can declare triumphantly that they have *scientifically proven* that Ashwagandha is incapable of curing the diseases, which alternative medicine supposedly speaks of being the right antidote and medicine?

So I also say, do not try any dosage of the medicine yourself, – any alternative medicine, including Ashwagandha or turmeric powder, internally, until you know the correct usage and the correct dosage.

Now let me give you one more example. In ancient times, a mother to be was given a Tonic to strengthen her and the baby, made up of Ashwagandha. The amount put in that tonic was 1 g of Ashwagandha root powder. I was shocked when I went online, and found out that some doctors were advocating tonics made of Ashwagandha and ginseng, as safe to expectant mothers, *irrespective of the dosage – 1 tablespoon.* Poor little baby. Poor little mother.

Notice the difference between 1 tablespoon and 1 g, which would be the equivalent of 1 teaspoon, which is 3 g. And here I am talking about 1 – 2 g which is never never taken raw. It is always mixed in milk, juice, or in any form, which dilutes the quantity, of the herb, and lessens the power of its strong qualities when it goes into the stomach.

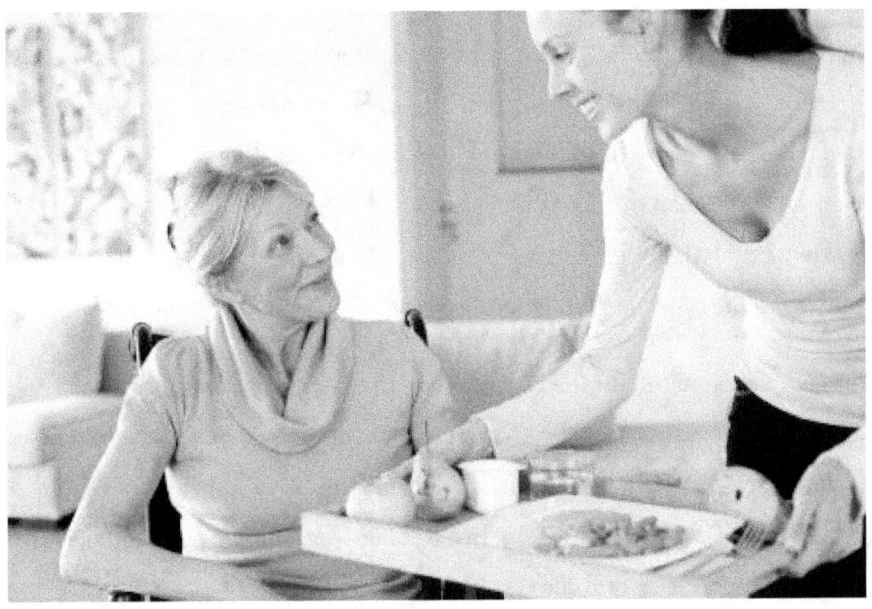

In ancient times, the elderly and the sick were given Ashwagandha in order to keep them healthy and to rejuvenate their tissues and muscles. Also, their bodies were massaged with Ashwagandha oil.

In ancient times, mothers to be were fed Ashwagandha powder in such tiny quantities in milk, and then after that they were fed, clarified butter, fruit and vegetables. The doctors of today with their incomplete knowledge, but because they have been "requested" by pharmaceutical companies to promote their products may tell you to take Ashwagandha in a tonic, – buy such and such brand-name – but they are not going to tell you about the diet you have to take in order to keep little baby healthy, and happy.

And then suddenly, the FDA or any researcher comes up with the horrifying news that Ashwagandha is harmful when taken by an expectant mother. Of course it is. If you are feeding her poison, how do you expect baby to get off scot- free?

So remember that all the recipes given here have been time-tested and are timeworn. They are traditional. You are not going to skimp on the quality of the ingredients being used by trying other substitutes like fruit juice concentrate instead of fresh fruit juice – when the recipe calls for it – or vegetable oil, when I am talking about clarified butter or when I say 2 g of Ashwagandha, you say, the more the merrier, and put in 2 tablespoons.

I am not accountable for the potentially harmful results of such irresponsible behavior. In small quantities, Ashwagandha was considered by people in ancient times, along with Emblica officianalis to be an extender of life and rejuvenator. That is why it was called a Rasa- yan or a natural element *Rasa* which extended the life force.

At that time, this particular plant was used to cure a number of ailments, including the diminishing powers of the brain, vitality, vigor, emaciation gynecological problems and disorders, rheumatism, inflammation, infections, immune diseases, and cough.

There is one reason why so many people in the world have become quite interested in this particular Herb today. That is because this is the natural equivalent of Viagra, and anybody who found his/her libido flagging – remember, this is a native of the land of the Kama Sutra – all they had to do was just go to their elders and ask for a tonic which would have them whole, healthy, and hearty again and ready for more sessions of Kama.

In fact, all the native vitality tonics sold by natural drug companies in Asia have ginseng and Ashwagandha in them. And I said before, there are some Japanese and American companies who are trying to take out patents for preparations made of this particular combination, especially when these tonics are going to be in the range of demand always exceeds supply, as long as human beings live, and obey their natural instincts.

In fact, the name says it all – ashwa-stallion – gandha- smell [possibly because the roots smelled strongly of horse sweat.] Also, this root was supposed to give you as much stamina and vitality, as would be expected in a healthy horse, and thus the name Ashwa – horse/stallion in Sanskrit.

Traditional uses of Ashwagandha

So how do you retain your good health and vitality with the passing of time?

Traditional remedies using Ashwagandha have come down through millenniums and the remedies in the book have been told to me by a natural medicine practitioner, well-versed in Ayurveda. In fact I was there, when he was preparing a bronchitis medicine for one of his patients with this root and clarified butter.

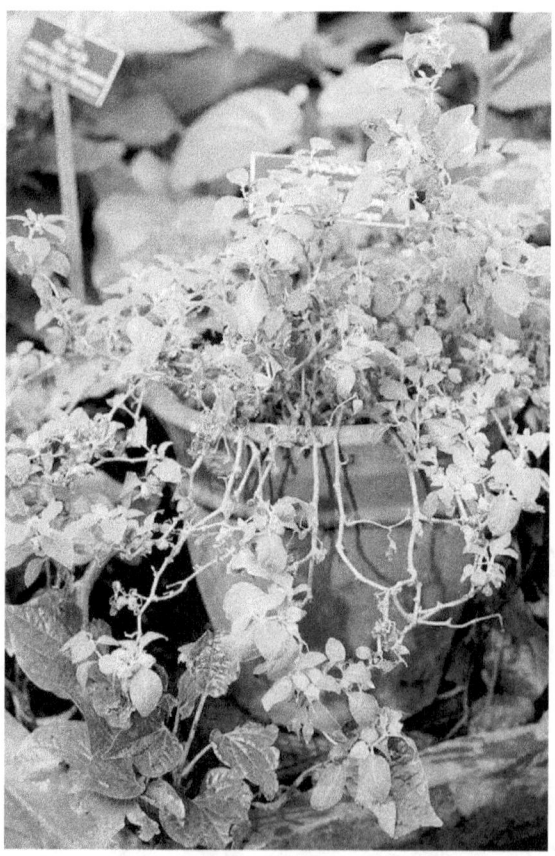

Cliff © <u>Wikimedia Commons</u>

Actually, Ashwagandha is one of the most popular of plants used in Ayurvedic medicine preparations, so thousands of tons of this plant is cultivated here.

It is a woody and small shrub, with little flowers, red fruit – seeds – and green leaves which are elliptical in shape. The green – yellowish flowers bloom throughout the year. The reason why this plant is so prolific, all over any tropical land, where there is plenty of water is because it is very hardy and it is going to survive in areas, where other plants wither and dry. That is because it has a really long taproot which can delve deep into the earth, in search of water. Along with that, it has a number of small side roots, and these are the precious parts of the plant.

You can get anywhere between 450 – 500 kilograms of fresh root in 1 acre of this cultivated plant. This is always dried, in the shade, so that you get around 125 – 150 kilograms of dehydrated root from about 500 kg of fresh root.

Calculate the usage in tons. Every year. Just in India. And now that Ashwagandha is being cultivated in Africa, America, and other parts of the world too, you can estimate the land needed to cultivate a plant. It is going to take one year in order to mature enough for harvesting. This harvesting is normally done in India, –no snow, harsh frost, or freezing cold in that particular area – from early January to late March. Also, incidentally, I found out that it grows very well, in areas, which is suffering from a drought condition, and if other plants do not survive, this plant is going to do so. Especially in the deserts/arid lands of South and central India and Rajasthan.

Growing Ashwagandha in Your Garden

This is a rather attractive plant, so if you want to grow it in your own garden. All you need is a container which can hold a plant which grows up to 3 feet. Within a year, you are going to have tiny attractive flowers looking like bells and followed with reddish orange berries.

Ashwagandha is normally planted through seeds, especially in the beginning of the rainy season in areas where the temperature is around 25 – 30°C. Like I said before, this can be grown in desert areas and arid lands, thus its extensive growth in Yemen and other parts of Africa.

The seeds are planted 10 cm from each other and 2 cm deep in the soil prepared with a rich organic fertilizer and well moistened with water. You are going to get germinated ceilings within 2 weeks. They are going to need plenty of water, while germinating and during their growth, but make sure that the soil does not get waterlogged. The temperature should be around 20°C or 70°F.

In a month's time, you are going to have enough plants, which can be thinned out, and you are going to do the thinning, leaving about 60 cm between plants, so that they have plenty of space to grow.

They like the sun. They also like an area which is dry. The soil has to be full of organic fertilizer. This is the reason why this plant grows best, wild where organic leaf compost in the woods has been piling up for centuries! Also, it likes soil which is sandy and well-drained, if the soil is slightly alkaline or neutral, this plant is going to flourish. The pH value should be around 8.

If the soil is waterlogged, you will not be able to grow Ashwagandha there. Incidentally, this plant grew wild in areas where there was less water in the wild, and that is why any watering that you do is going to be done only when you feel that the soil is totally dry, cracked, and it needs just that much water in order to survive. Better drought than overwatering.

If the temperature is above or below 20° – 35°C, you are going to find the plant growing even more slowly.

You are not going to put any chemical fertilizer near this plant, because its power is in its roots. However, when you are applying natural organic fertilizers, you are going to place that fertilizer away from the stem of the plant, but near enough so that the nutrients can go into the soil.

If you are growing Ashwagandha in a cold climate, bring your plants indoors at the first hint of frost. Basically, it is a spring/summer plant, so plant it and harvest it before the coming of the winter.

Harvesting Time

The moment you see the red berries and the leaves beginning to dry out, within 6 months of sowing, it is time to harvest your roots. You are going to wet the soil around the plant and do the digging very carefully with a small tool, taking care not to harm the roots. These roots are then washed clean of all the debris after they have been cut from the main plant stem.

Now you are going to cut these roots into pieces of 10 cm and dry them in the shade. So now you have lots of precious dried Ashwagandha root.

The berries are also gathered, and dried, so that the seeds can be taken for other medicinal preparations.

Traditional Preparation for Restoring Vitality and Vigor

A traditional Ayurvedic formula, which was told to me by one of the traditional herbalists – to restore flagging vitality, especially for people who wanted their sexual stamina to be restored – is given here.

Remember, that this herb is not to be taken indiscriminately, especially for people, who think that taking an herb in large quantities is going to make them virile and strong. Along with it, you have to look at your diet.

Remember that millenniums ago, when people use to eat herbs in order to restore themselves physically, and mentally, they also made sure that the rest of their diet was healthy and pure. That is why they ate and drank plenty of milk products, drank fresh buttermilk, with lots of homemade butter, and clarified butter.

In fact, it has been written in the Bible that the great Wise men, leaders of men and prophets considered homemade butter to be the reason why they could have and raise strong sons, and also the reason for their own longevity and fertility. It is a proven fact, and you do not need to spend billions of dollars on researching this already time-tested and timeworn proven matter. This was in the biblical lands.

Well, let me tell you one secret. This recipe was known to every earthy and red-blooded woman in ancient India, especially one who enjoyed the pleasures of her marital bed with her husband, – who she referred to in the village as her "Bull."

This may sound very barbaric to a much more civilized people, especially when we do not talk very freely about natural instincts, and our repressed, over civilized 21st century world, but in ancient times and in ancient civilizations, women liked to boast about the prowess of their men in keeping their women satisfied and happy, and also bearing lots and lots of healthy children.

Whenever they found their husbands, saying, "not tonight, Josephine, I have a headache," they immediately gathered this herb, got out their clarified butter, and prepared this restorative.

They used just 10 g of this very powerful mixture in 125 g of hot milk with a spoonful of honey, and fed it to him after dinner. And then the next morning, they would go boasting to all their friends that their man was a real he-man, worthy to be the fit mate and husband of a real Earth mother goddess she – woman.

Incidentally, this boasting is not restricted to just women in the East. I have heard the same terms being used by women in Greece, Spain, Egypt, Italy, South America, and other women, belonging to ancient civilizations, even today!

But never in Britain, where this sort of talk is considered heathenish barbaric, rude, crude, and definitely not civilized, and not quite ladylike.

That was because the British, down the ages had started to consider sex as something not to be spoken about, and sinful, and shameful – especially in the Middle Ages – those dark ages – and especially in Victorian times, when mothers told their daughters about to get married that they had to bear the travails of the marriage bed, and well, they just had to think that childbearing had to be done for the good of England.

And if they were lucky, they would be left alone, and their husbands could enjoy this sport with their mistresses. No wonder they were so repressed, ignorant, and ill-informed of natural processes and went around the world with their ideas of natural human instincts being something not quite so nice and definitely not something to be encouraged.

So the idea of any sort of aphrodisiac, especially which was used as a traditional medicine in the East, would not have been accepted in the family medicine cabinet, because it was something which the "eastern barbarians" used, in order to have lots and lots of children. Or perhaps the passionate people of the Mediterranean countries like Italy and Spain, but definitely not the British!

And their mamas had told them that any sort of enjoyment in the marriage bed was sinful, was unnatural, and definitely not something to be encouraged. And for thousands of years, this one little island held onto this belief, and spread it all over the world. Any woman who was red-blooded and enjoyed her natural instincts was called wicked, sinful, a Jezebel, and promiscuous.

And that is why Henry VIII's redheaded hot blooded daughter with all her "favorites" and "friends" declared herself the Virgin Queen, in a tongue-in-cheek way, and the Britishers would believe it to be so when the whole world knows *it ain't necessarily so*!

Naturally, this traditional Eastern aphrodisiac is not for people, who shrink at the idea of natural basic instincts, but still go around looking for any sort of alternatives to prove to themselves, they are still youthfully vigorous. Thus, the continual demand for Viagra and Cialis.

But as we are talking about an Herb from the East, the Indian ginseng, like all ancient civilizations, this herbal preparation was also made in a concentrated powerful butter base. For this you are going to need clarified butter.

Incidentally, this is one basic preparation, which you are going to use to cure bronchitis, asthma, and also restore yourself to vitality – depending on the amount I tell you to take, along with how many times you take it, and with how much milk.

You take 250 g of *Nagori Ashwagandha* root- this is the traditional real ancient name of this root. It means that it has been harvested wild.

You are going to take 250 g of dried ginger root which has been crushed, pounded into a powder in a pestle and mortar and filtered.

Now take four ladles of pure clarified butter in order to fry this mixture until it is dark brown in color.

Now you are going to take 250 g of *desi khand*. (Literally – "native/local sugar". This is sugarcane unrefined pure sugar, and it has been used for centuries to prepare Ayurvedic medicines, because of the power of sugarcane as a restorative.) Do not worry; I am going to tell you where you can get these ingredients on line and in their pure form.[1]

---

[1] Desi Khand-

http://www.swadeshaj.com/natural-sweeteners/394-deshi-khand.html

You may want to contact them and ask them whether they ship abroad. The price given here (Rs 60) is equivalent to a dollar, and 3 times the price of ordinary sugar, which is priced around $0.20 – $0.30 locally! This is also called Khand sari- (kh-uhnd-saari-) meaning – just pure concentrated sugar.

Incidentally, I did not know about that artificial sweetener Aspartame, the bane of the FDA. So here is one instructive and interesting URL, telling you how a sweet lobby is trying its best to feed you poisons like refined sugar, corn syrup and

Add the sugar to the brown fried mixture, and just enough water, frying continuously, on low heat until the clarified butter rises to the surface. This means that everything has been cooked properly.

So remember, you are just going to take 10 g of this powerful mixture in 125 g of milk in this particular instance.

For asthma and bronchitis, the remedy is given below, even though the preparation procedure using clarified butter is the same.

---

aspartame and discouraging the consumption of natural healthy traditional sweet sources.

– http://www.educationworldonline.net/index.php/page-article-choice-more-id-248

Ashwagandha-

http://www.ebay.com/itm/Ashwagandha-Roots-Withania-Somnifera-Indian-Raw-Whole-Herbs-/281239000837?var=&hash=item417b269705:m:mgf0oaoYWtNTT2zasGDroAA

Preparing Clarified Butter

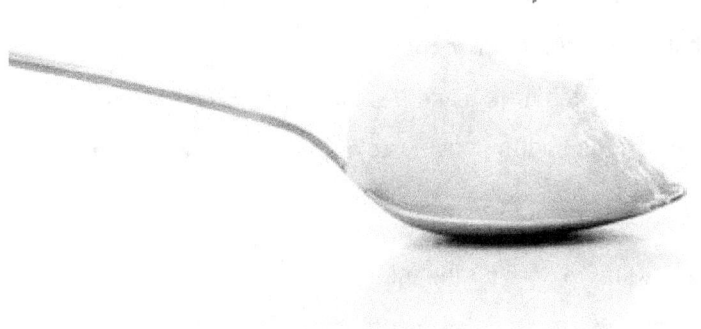

You are not going to buy clarified butter, because it turns out to be a really expensive proposition, unless you have lots of butter, ready at hand from your own dairy farm!

Instead, you are going to make it at home with this instructive URL –

https://www.youtube.com/watch?v=aF_tdNwqvKQ

The idea of buying clarified butter from the market is an anathema maranatha for any house proud Eastern Cook.

This is my way.

You make this at home by taking 2 pounds of best unsalted butter and melting it in a heavy bottomed pan. Allow the butter to liquefy on low heat for about 40 minutes. Maintain this simmering point, until all of the moisture in the butter has evaporated. The impurities are going to sink to the bottom of the pan. Remember to keep stirring the butter, so that it does not burn.

Pour off the clear butter and strain it through several thicknesses of muslin cloth. This butter is going to last for about a year, if it is placed in a cool and dry place. This butter is exorbitantly expensive. So in the East, people with easy access to plenty of fresh milk make it right in their kitchens for crisp delicious frying results, and adding that taste of pure butter to all their dishes.

Also, what are you going to do with the impurities? Do not throw them away or discard them, because they are really delicious, when heated a little and mixed with molasses. Spread all over your toasted bread and eat.

Clarified butter is highly concentrated. That is why it is a bit difficult to digest, when eaten on its own. However, as it is a staple for giving and nourishing of the elderly, it is always mixed up in their vegetables, meat, or beans so that it is easier to digest.

Recognizing Pure Clarified Butter

So how are you going to recognize pure clarified butter, especially when you go to a shop, and ask for butter oil or clarified butter or ghee? Here is the traditional way in which you can find, if the butter has been adulterated with any other oil product or milk products.

Pick up a dried clay pot or utensil and rub some clarified butter on the surface. After a while, if you see a layer of white, where they should be absolutely no layer, which means it has been adulterated.

Another method is to take a glass bowl, and add a little bit of mustard oil to it. Now add a little bit of this clarified butter which you bought from the market to it, if there is any adulteration and the clarified butter is not hundred percent pure, it is going to float on the surface of the mustard oil. However, if it is pure, it is going to sink right to the bottom of the glass bowl.

When I told all my friends these two time-tested methods in nodded to take up the purity of clarified butter, they went around making the lives of all the shopkeepers in the vicinity miserable by asking for a test done immediately. And being quite bossy type of voluble ladies, they managed to entertain the whole market, especially when they asked for some of the well-known Agro dairy companies' clarified butter products to be tested then and there.

In fact, one poor beleaguered shopkeeper requested them to go grab hold of those particular companies' top people's throats, instead of shouting at him; he was just the innocent bystander, selling their products! This supposedly very expensive clarified butter is often made up of a mixture of different vegetable oils, to which the essence of clarified butter is mixed and then packaged and sold as one hundred percent clarified butter.

Traditional Bronchitis and Asthma Cure

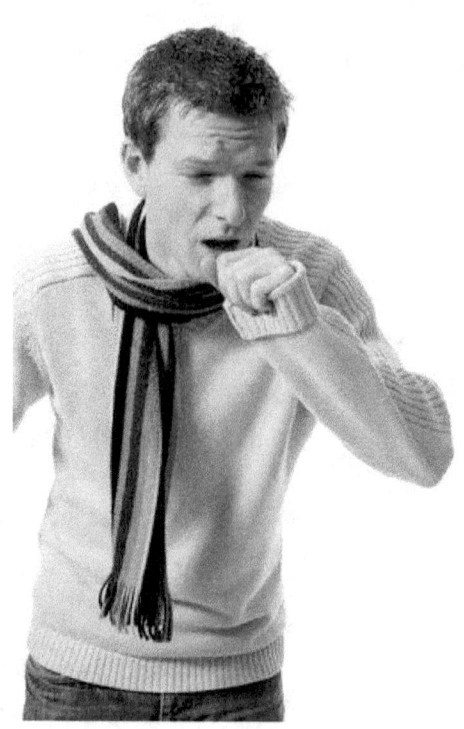

Believe it or not, this cure has been used for centuries to cure chronic bronchitis and asthma *within 10 days,* 15 days at the most in more serious chronic cases. Impossible, you say. You have been spending so much money on your bronchitis and asthma drugs, and according to your doctors, these are conditions which can only be controlled and not cured.

Well, take my word for it. Try this remedy.

Take 250 g of Aswagandha in desi ghee – clarified butter. You are not going to be using dried ginger here , but you are going to be using the above given method to make a fried desi ghee- aswagandha mixture to make up a mixture. This has to be drunk with milk once a day until the bronchitis/ asthma is cured. You are going to take 2 tablespoons full of this mixture in one glass of hot milk. To this, you are going to add one tablespoonful of honey. Drink it down fast, and go to sleep, with a cotton bedsheet covering your body. This mixture taken just before you go to sleep can also cure insomnia.

Another traditional aphrodisiac remedy taken from the ancient texts was made with one part of Ashwagandha root with one part of clarified butter and 10 parts of milk. This was boiled down slowly and steadily until all the milk was evaporated and only the clarified butter was left.

Even today, this Ayurvedic preparation is sold extensively, all over India in the form of Ashwagandha ghee. You take a heaped tablespoon in the morning and in the evening with a glass of warm milk. And you do not have to worry about Viagra, Cialis, or any other 21st-century modern-day equivalents.

Incidentally, for ages Ashwagandha root has been used to enhance clarity of thought, brainpower, reduce stress, strain, and strengthen your immune system.

Now let me tell you the scientific reason why this particular root is supposed to be such an enhancer of your libido. The answer is very simple; it has a natural adaptogen which relaxes the stress creating factors in your brain. Once you find yourself getting less stressed, you are going to feel all your systems feeling stronger, and more vigorous.

So naturally, when you do not feel stressed out, you immediately feel a rise in your natural libido and that is because like in other parts of your body, your glands have been stimulated de stressed and revitalized, you are going to find the same positive and beneficial effect affecting your natural basic instincts too. Simple explanation!

Remember, if you are using the powdered root, which you are buying in America, in the drug supplement market, make sure that you do not take more than one teaspoonful at one time. **That is 3 g. And this is going to be in a glass full of milk. If you are taking 2 teaspoons full – 6 g, – twice a day, make sure that you have at least an interval of 8 hours, before you take these 2 doses. Like morning and evening.**

Nowadays, you can get a number of companies, giving you an extract of Ashwagandha which has about 500 mg of Ashwagandha extract. It is in concentrated form, and I am not quite sure about how many fillers have gone into the making up of that particular capsule. But there are about 5% of withanolides in one capsule, when compared to hundred percent of the natural product in a natural preparation.

Incidentally, as this plant belongs to the nightshade family, you can call it a younger brother of the deadly nightshade. It is also called winter cherry or even poison gooseberry. Somnifera means sleep inducing, and once upon a time, this root in small quantities was given to patients, in order to induce sleep. That is why, people suffering from chronic insomnia are given a number of tonics with a little bit of Ashwagandha powder in it.

So you want to know whether you can grow Ashwagandha in your own climate? Well, if there are tomatoes growing in your garden and lots of them, you can also grow Ashwagandha! That is because both of them belong to the same family, Solanaceae.

Remember that you are never going to use this particular Herb, when you are using barbiturates – with the recommended to you by your doctor or just eaten through a habit. This increases the power and potency of barbiturates, because both are sleep inducing. Incidentally, you are not going to take this particular Herb, if you are suffering from any sort of respiratory problem or suffer from natural congestion.

Ashwagandha for Rejuvenation

Here is the rejuvenative restorative formula taken from ancient texts.

You are going to use Ashwagandha and clarified butter, honey, and long pepper –pippali in the ratio of 10: 10:5:1. [5 parts of honey and one part of long pepper.]

Pippali – long pepper – is a rejuvenating spice which has not found its way into many Western kitchens yet, and you can get to know more about it on this URL.

https://en.wikipedia.org/wiki/Long_pepper

Before its use as a spice, it was used as a curative healing agent.[2] you are going to grind them all together and put them in a glass jar. You are going to take one teaspoonful of this mixture, once a day, either at breakfast with a glass full of milk, or before you go to sleep with a glass full of milk, so that you can stay healthy, young and rejuvenated throughout your life.

Incidentally, this plant is not restricted to the Indian subcontinent. You can find it in Yemen, parts of Africa, China, and other parts of Asia too. In

---

[2] http://www.ebay.in/itm/Long-Pepper-Piper-Longum-Dried-Catkins-Pippali-Herbal-Powder-50g-/390754532830

This seller seems to have powdered Long Pepper. I would suggest buying the spice whole, and powdering it yourself. There must be other places where you could get it in its original form and at a more economical rate.

If you can get it at your local herbs store, if you cannot get it under the name of long Pepper, ask for pipp- uhlly- (Pippalli.). The shopkeeper is going to say, "you want pepper?" No, you are going to say , *"you want long pepper."* Ordinary pepper is small and rounded peppercorns. Pippali are long catkins.

Yemen, where it is called ubab – these berries are used by people who do not have access to rennet when they are making cheese.

In fact, if you are traveling in Africa, and you find yourself wounded and there is Ashwagandha around, all you have to do is collect some of the leaves, berries, and make them into a paste. Apply the paste on the wounds to prevent infection. This remedy is also good for curing burns. In other parts of the world, the leaves and the berries were pounded together, into a paste, and applied on boils, carbuncles, and even tumors to cure them.

Ashwagandha Massage Oil

Incidentally, this is one recipe, which can be taken internally because we are using an Ashwagandha decoction in clarified butter. It is tasty and healthy. It can also be used externally as a massage oil, especially when your skin is dry, or you want your skin to look healthy, youthful and full of a young glow.

For this, you are going to need one litre of pure spring water without any impurities, or chlorine additives. In ancient times, you had plenty of this water around in order to make decoctions, but today you have to hunt for it!

To this, you are going to add 8 tablespoons – 2 ounces of Ashwagandha powder. You are going to heat this on medium heat, until the mixture is reduced to one fourth of the quantity. This is going to take anywhere between 45 minutes to one hour. This is going to be filtered and strained through a fine muslin cloth and this is the valuable Ashwagandha concentrated decoction. Allow it to cool. Now take 8 ounces of pure clarified butter and place it on heat, adding the decoction to this mixture.

Heat slowly, stirring frequently for about 2 hours, until all the water has boiled off.

This is now your valuable powerful oil to be used externally as a massage oil, if you want to strengthen the muscles and give the tissues proper restorative power and also as an internal strengthening tonic, of which you are going to take just one teaspoon with your dinner and one teaspoon for lunch – never more than 2 teaspoons in one day – spread on any gravy, meat, or anything else of which you want to improve the taste!

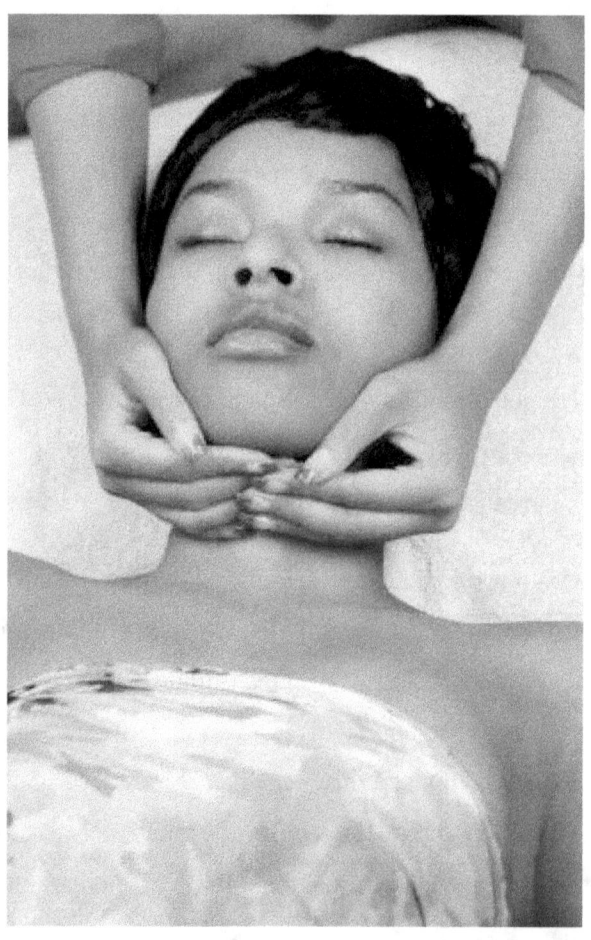

Incidentally, in ancient times, if a child was weak, and did not show a healthy tissue growth, his grandmother would massage him with this particular massage oil 3 – 10 drops, depending on how old he was – 3 – 4 drops for babies and 6 drops for youngsters, 10 drops for adults – and also feed him food or bread on which this fortified clarified butter. Within 6 months that boy would be healthy, hearty, strong, and a kid to gladden his grandma's heart! And then she would put a black dot of soot on his face in order to ward off the evil eye!

Along with that, it is going to increase the body weight of that emaciated and thin baby, encourage tissue growth and give them plenty of energy and strength.

Get Rid of That Sweet Tooth!

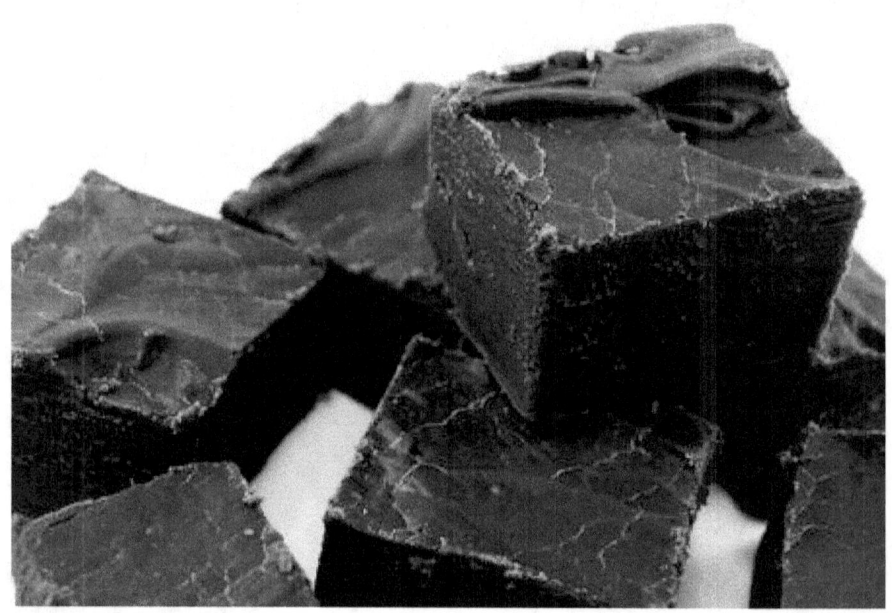

Unfortunately, many people are suffering from a sugar addiction. It is almost as powerful a health affecting factor as is a drug addiction or an alcohol addiction, but your doctor is never going to tell you that. Nor is the sugar lobby, which keeps tempting you to eat more and more sugar-based products.

Incidentally, in Ayurveda, eating something sweet in large quantities – they knew of what they spoke – was not considered to be healthy, and even though doctors know all about this sweet addiction, which is as dangerous as an addiction to alcohol, caffeine, and even nicotine, but who is there to tell you that all the foods out there that you eat, with plenty of corn syrup, and other sweet derivatives like aspartame and artificial sugar are definitely not good for your health.

So try the ancient way in which you can get rid of this craving for sweet foods. Take just enough clarified butter in which you can roast an ounce of Ashwagandha root. Fry it until it is golden brown. To this, you are going to add 1 tablespoon full of date sugar. Remember, that this is a traditional Yemen recipe, and date sugar was the traditional sugar made down the centuries to sweeten their delicious dishes. Naturally, people began craving sweets. Once you have made up this mixture, you are going to store it in an airtight glass jar.

You are just going to take half a teaspoonful of this mixture, with a cup of milk, whenever you want something sweet to eat. You can also eat this mixture, instead of something sweet half an hour before you have your breakfast. You are soon going to find yourself weaned away from a craving for something sweet *at* all times of the day. You can preserve this in the refrigerator until you finish this up and make the next batch.

This is because the Ashwagandha is capable of restoring the tissues of the brain and its bio physiological activities in a natural manner to prevent the craving of sweets. Incidentally, this is a healthy alternative to all those artificial sugar laden foods found on your supermarket shelves today.

Ashwagandha for Reducing Cholesterol Levels

Try one teaspoonful of Ashwagandha powder, once a day, boiled in a glass full of milk. If your cholesterol level is really high, you are going to have one teaspoonful – 3 grams – in milk once in the morning and once in the evening. It is also good for reducing the levels of blood sugar for diabetics.

Side Effects of Ashwagandha

Everything in excess is not good for your health, so even though in the East, this is given as a rejuvenating tonic to expectant mothers, in the West, it is supposed to cause miscarriages. This is because doctors prescribe excessive doses of this herb, without even thinking of the harmful side effects and with an incomplete knowledge of this particular Herb. So if you are expecting and you do not have an experienced herbalist around, do not take Ashwagandha.

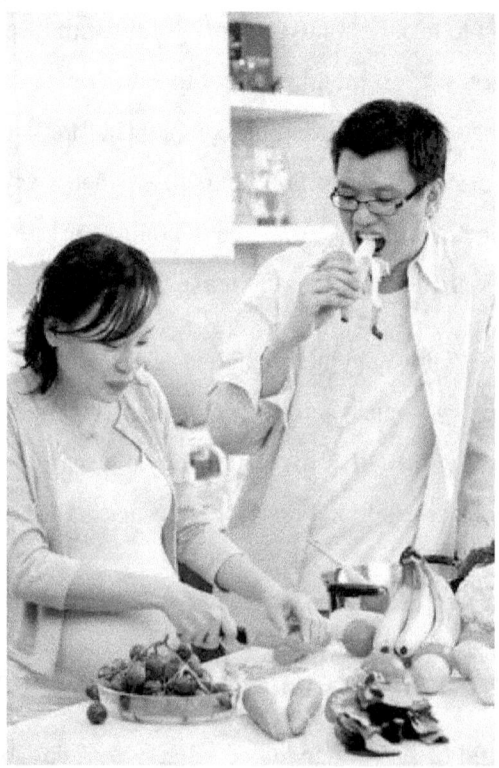

This expecting mother knows all about a healthy diet for the good of her family, and baby.

Also, if you are suffering from vomiting and diarrhea, which means you have been taking this herb in large quantities. PLEASE STOP THAT IMMEDIATELY. Do not try any experiments with your health, just thinking that taking more of something will have a more powerful effect on your system.

Conclusion

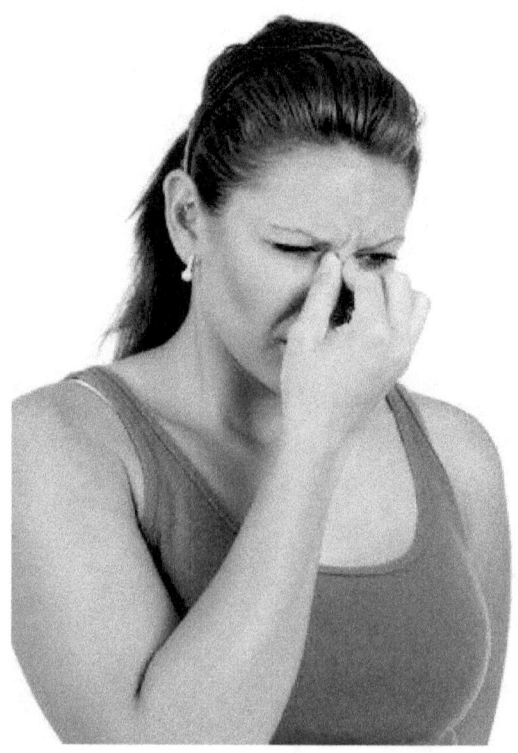

Stressed, nervous, think your life is full of tension? Do a little bit of natural relaxing with natural remedies like Ashwagandha.

I have now introduced you to a new herb, Ashwagandha, and how you can use it. Naturally, if you have been reading through other books in my herb and spices series, you are going to notice that often I go into a possibly frantic and frenzied diatribe against products made of chemical preservatives, artificial fillers, and other chemical-based products, taking the place of natural foods, herbs, spices and other healing natural bounties of nature.

So this book is telling you how you can use Ashwagandha as rejuvenating, as well as healing herb while also leading you to information about a chemical-based modern-day poison known as aspartame or as an artificial sweetener.

Just imagine that you are in a situation where everything has been destroyed in a cataclysm and you have no access to medicines, drugs, and other 21st-century boons, like ready to eat canned food, supplements, and other things which you have been brainwashed into thinking are all that are keeping you healthy and alive, and one step away from total debilitation.

This is when you are going to need the knowledge of the ages, which is going to be in the form of natural plants, foods, fruit, herbs, seeds, and if you know how to survive on these plants while gathering enough good for your family and tribe, well, you have managed to show the natural human instinct of survival is a state of mind.

So, here is the knowledge of the ages, coming down to you and not being spoon-fed to you, through doctors and researchers giving you incomplete and harmful knowledge with the support of pharmaceutical lobbies and brands. Remember that nature has given many good things to you, and the knowledge is out there. All you have to do is learn from the ancients, who have tested out these remedies, their dosage, and usage, for the benefit of mankind all over the world. Those ancients never intended you to be benefited temporarily through remedies which would remove one particular malady and gave rise to another malady through their medicines, as an accompanying side effect.

Unfortunately, all the medicines that you eat today are going to give you temporary relief. They are also going to have a number of side effects, which are not going to be told to you by your doctor. And then you are going to get stressed out when you see that horrible huge scary medical bill for an ailment, which would have gone away on its own, if you had not gone to the doctor, who immediately prescribed lots and lots and lots of expensive procedures and tests and medical drugs in order to get rid of a common cold.

And then you get so stressed out. You do not know what to do. So you take some prescribed medicines which do not seem to have a long-term effect on you, even though they have given you temporary relief.

The medicines from the ancients' cornucopia of knowledge, however, were one hundred percent natural, and they made sure that the ailment was cured permanently. They did not give you a medicine which would cure your cold, but gave rise to bronchitis instead because it had destroyed your immunity system.

So remember, nature is the best healer. She is the best provider of natural medicines. And best of all her medicines are available all over the earth, along with the healing remedies, somewhere out there, written by the ancients for me, for you and for little Tawny and Sonsie in Paraburdoo.

I am trying my little best in order to spread this knowledge to one and all, as far as I am able, especially because having lived in the lap of nature, all over the compass in woods, mountains, and jungles of inaccessible areas, for the first 16 years of my life, before I went to College in a small city, I am a 100% believer in no drugs, no chemical-based medicines, no hospitals, and leaving it all to nature and a natural healthy immunity system.

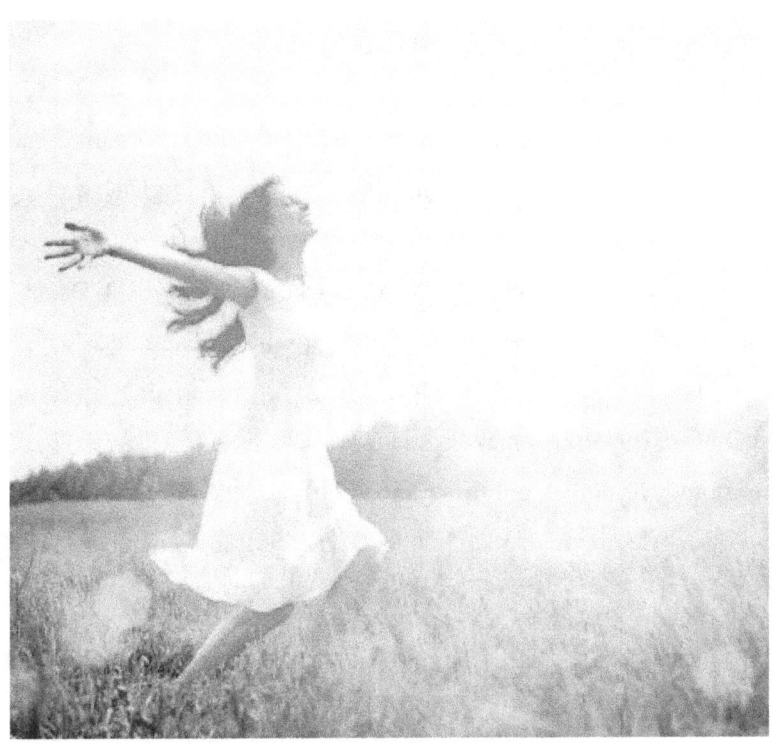

Life is good! Give ye thanks for all that you have been given.

You can also have that by just changing your lifestyle and getting back to a natural way of living.

So give thanks for and to Mother nature, Live Long and Prosper!

Author Bio

Dueep Jyot Singh is a Management and IT Professional who managed to gather Postgraduate qualifications in Management and English and Degrees in Science, French and Education while pursuing different enjoyable career options like being an hospital administrator, IT,SEO and HRD Database Manager/ trainer, movie , radio and TV scriptwriter, theatre artiste and public speaker, lecturer in French, Marketing and Advertising, ex-Editor of Hearts On Fire (now known as Solstice) Books Missouri USA, advice columnist and cartoonist, publisher and Aviation School trainer, ex-moderator on Medico.in, banker, student councilor ,travelogue writer … among other things!

One fine morning, she decided that she had enough of killing herself by Degrees and went back to her first love -- writing. It's more enjoyable! She already has 48 published academic and 14 fiction- in- different- genre books under her belt.

When she is not designing websites or making Graphic design illustrations for clients , she is browsing through old bookshops hunting for treasures, of which she has an enviable collection – including R.L. Stevenson, O.Henry, Dornford Yates, Maurice Walsh, De Maupassant, Victor Hugo, Sapper, C.N. Williamson, "Bartimeus" and the crown of her collection- Dickens "The Old Curiosity Shop," and "Martin Chuzzlewit" and so on… Just call her "Renaissance Woman" - collecting herbal remedies, acting like Universal Helping Hand/Agony Aunt, or escaping to her dear mountains for a bit of exploring, collecting herbs and plants, and trekking.

Check out some of the other JD-Biz Publishing books

Gardening Series on Amazon

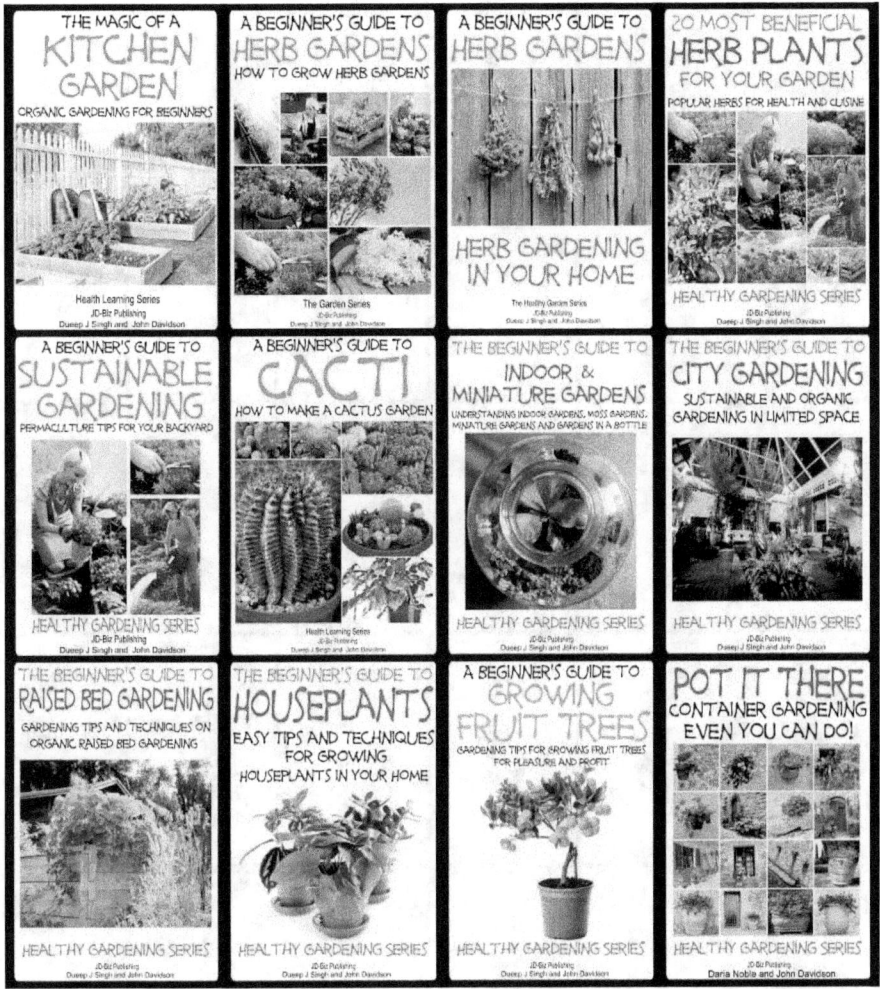

Download Free Books!

http://MendonCottageBooks.com

Health Learning Series

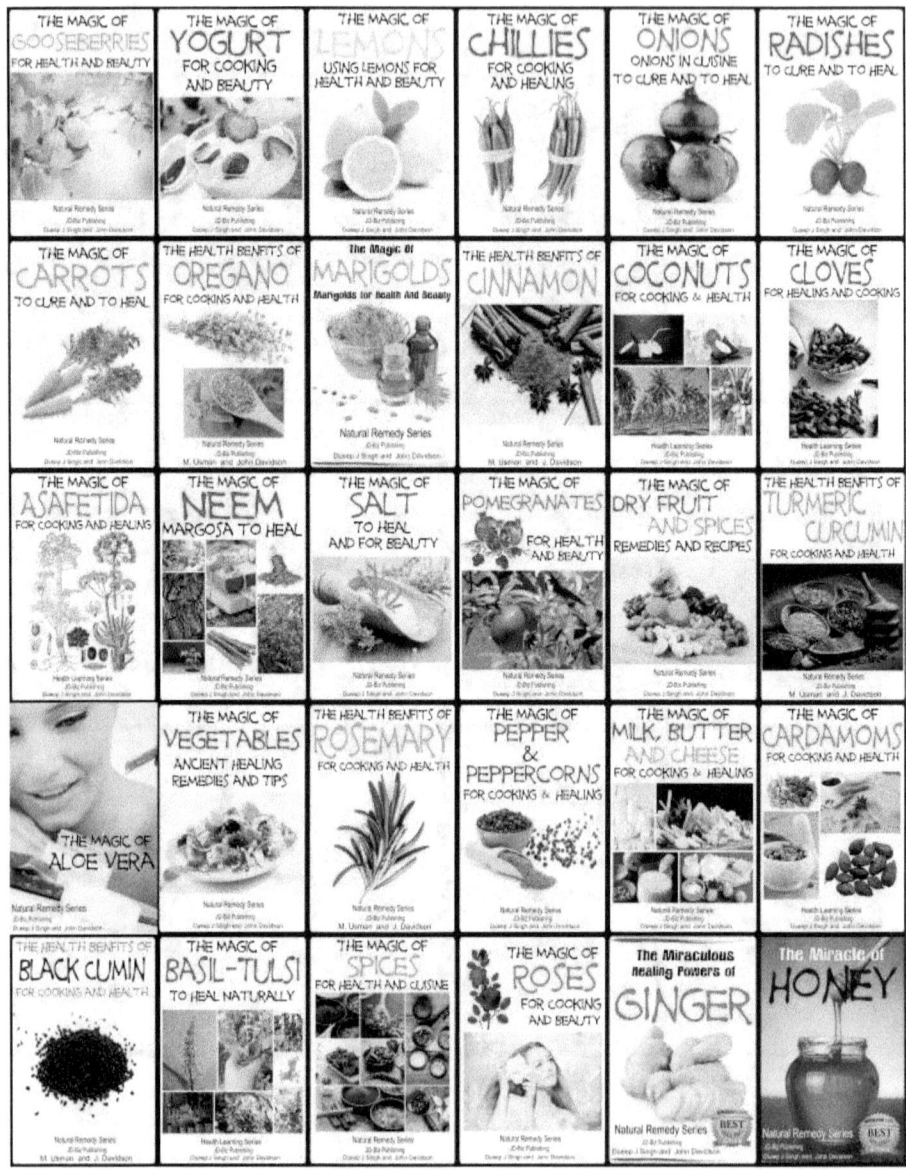

Country Life Books

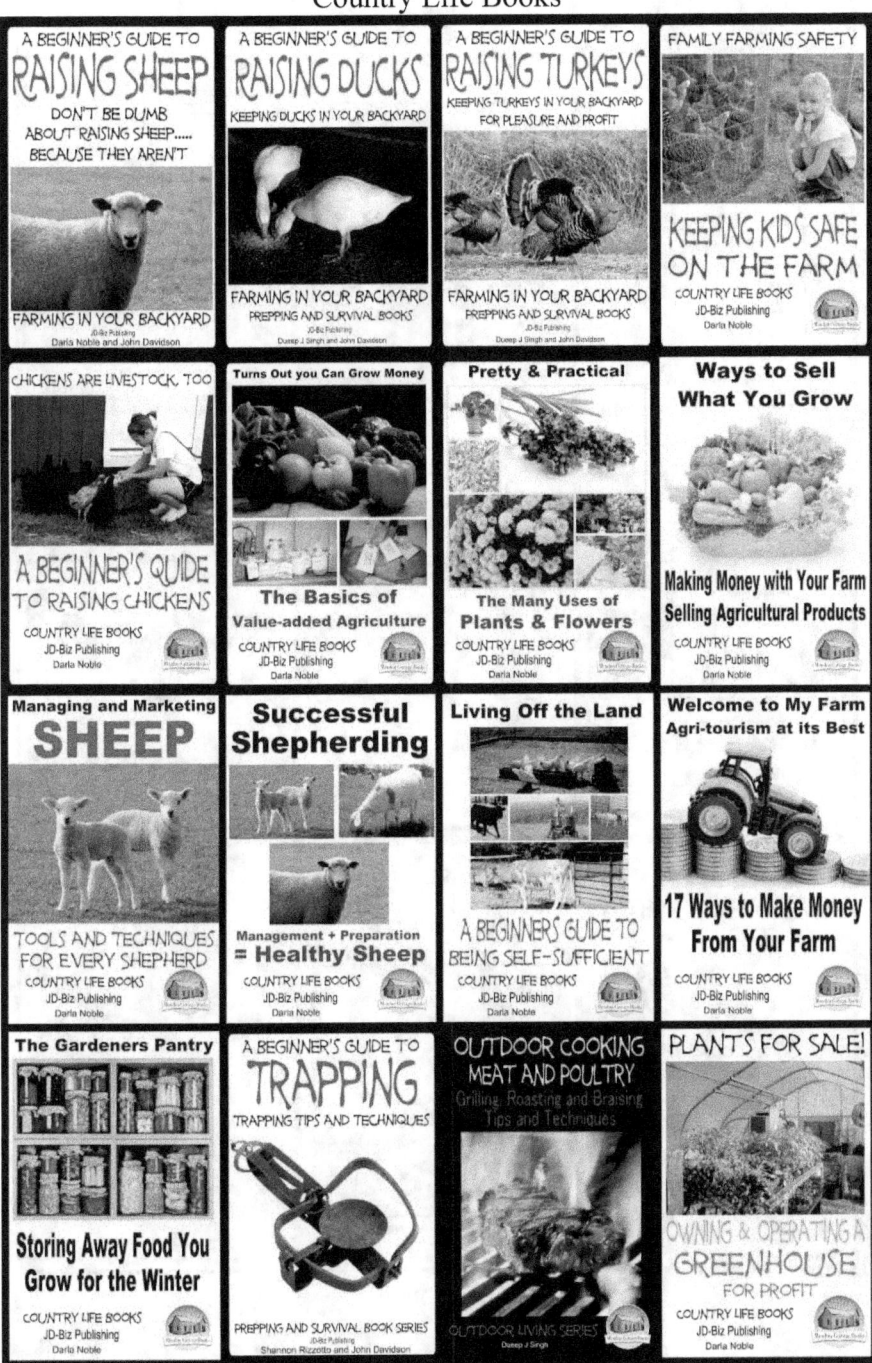

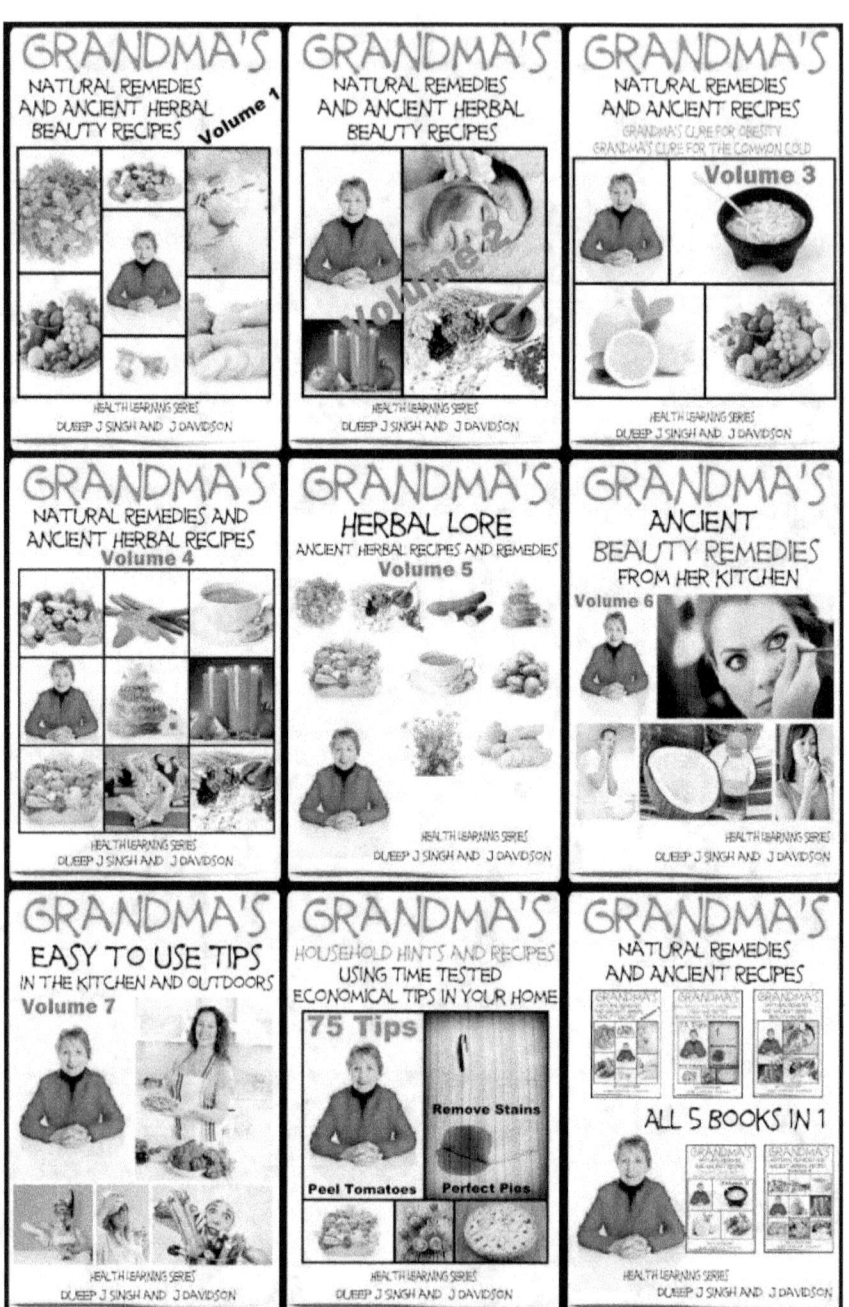

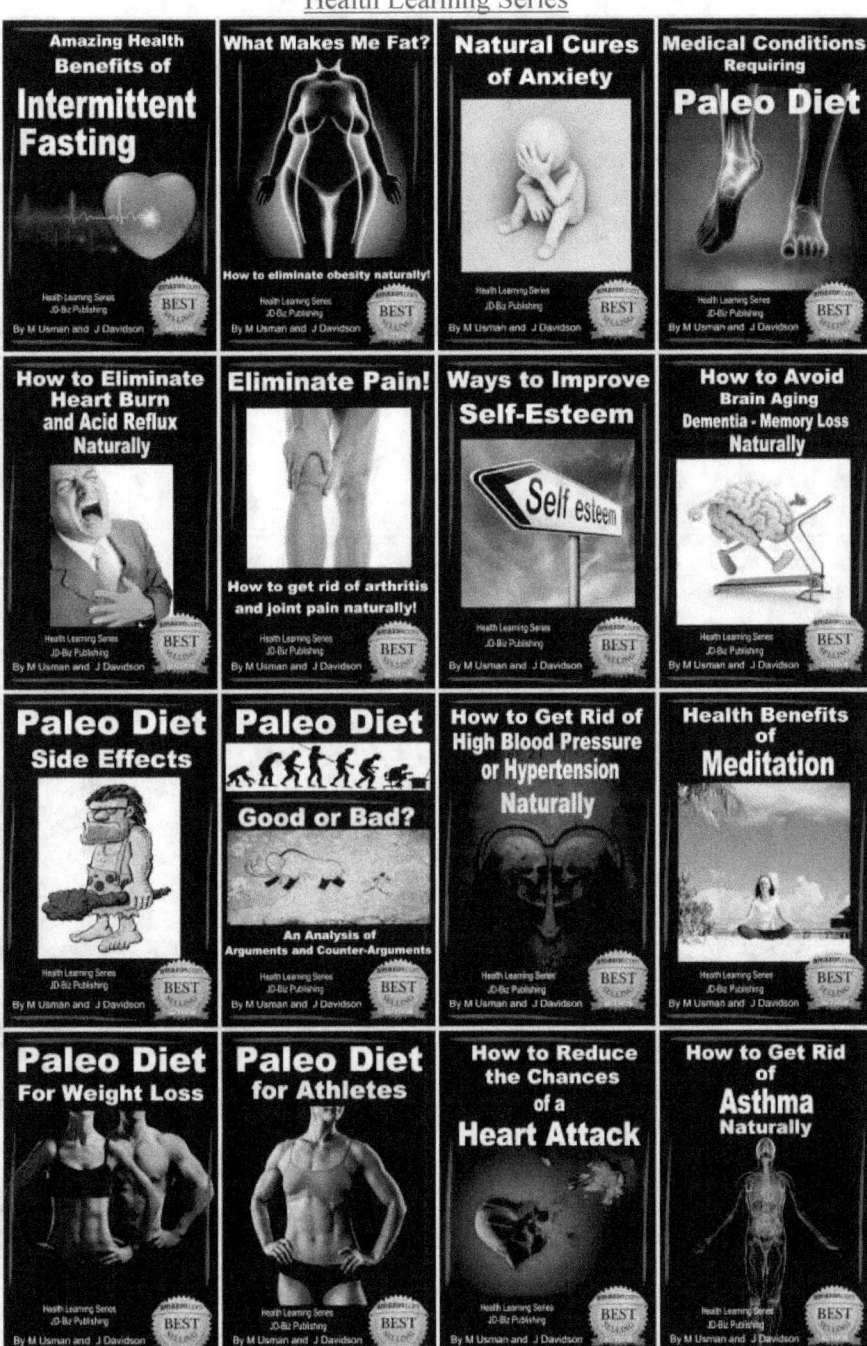

Amazing Animal Book Series

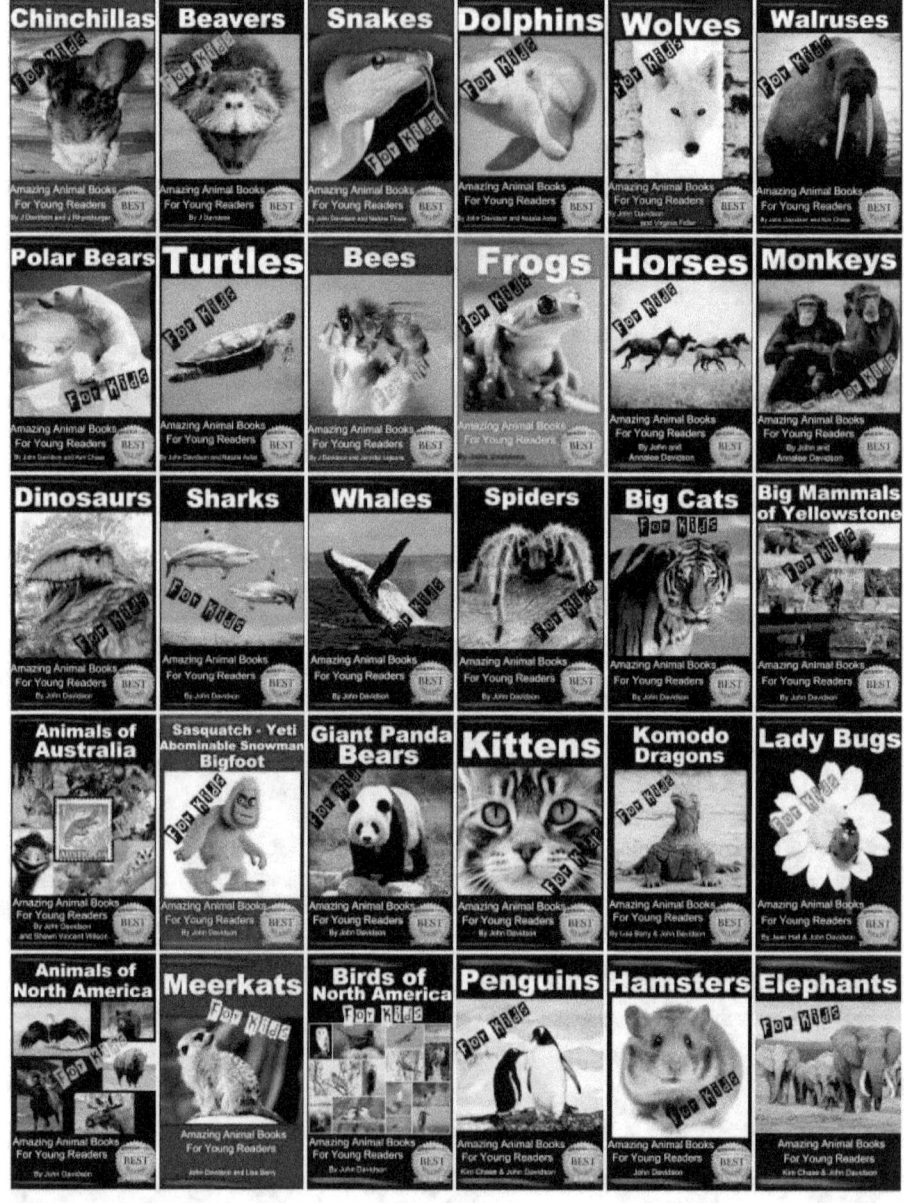

Learn To Draw Series

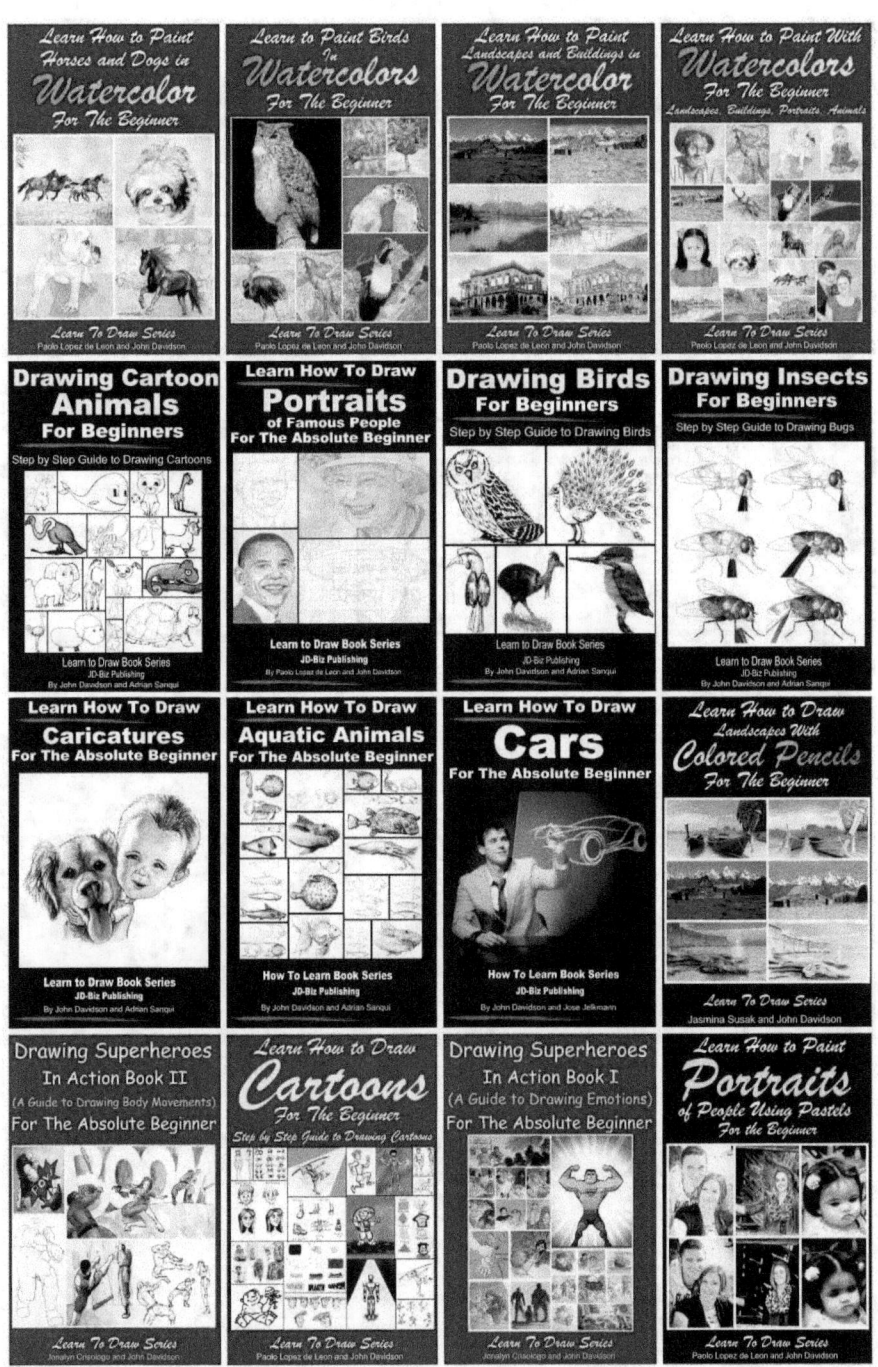

How to Build and Plan Books

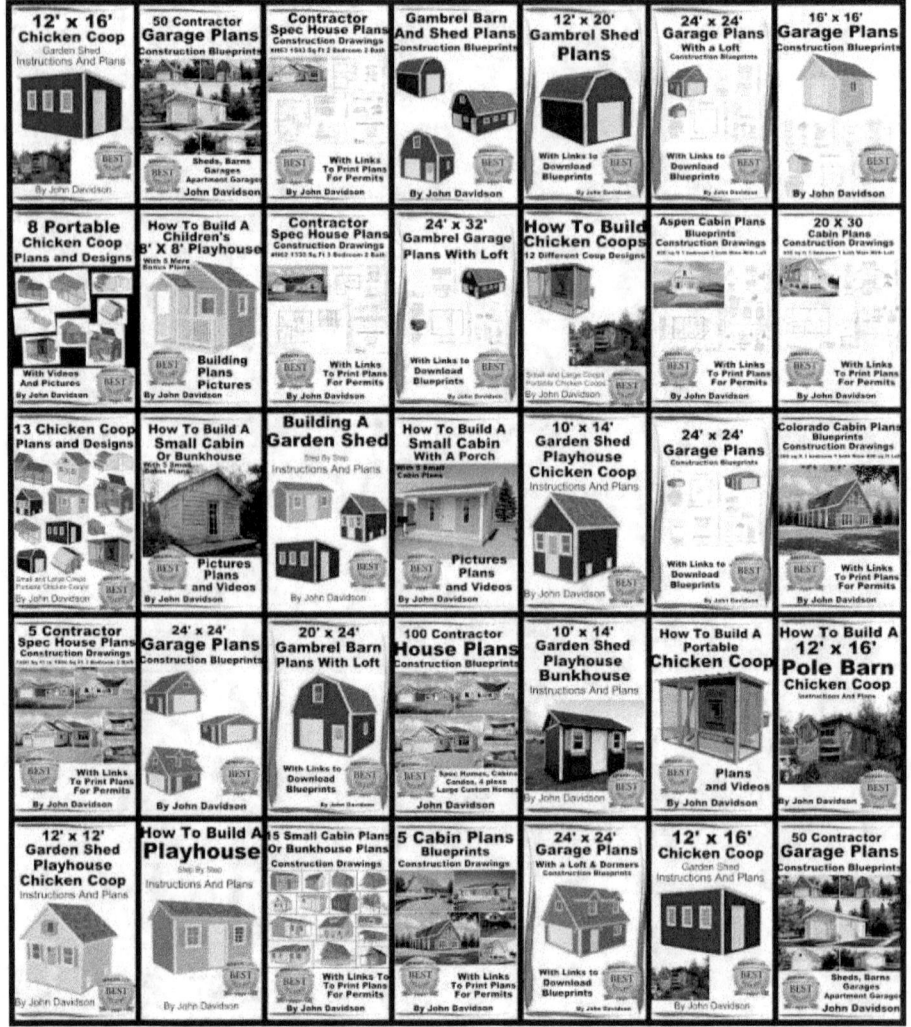

Entrepreneur Book Series

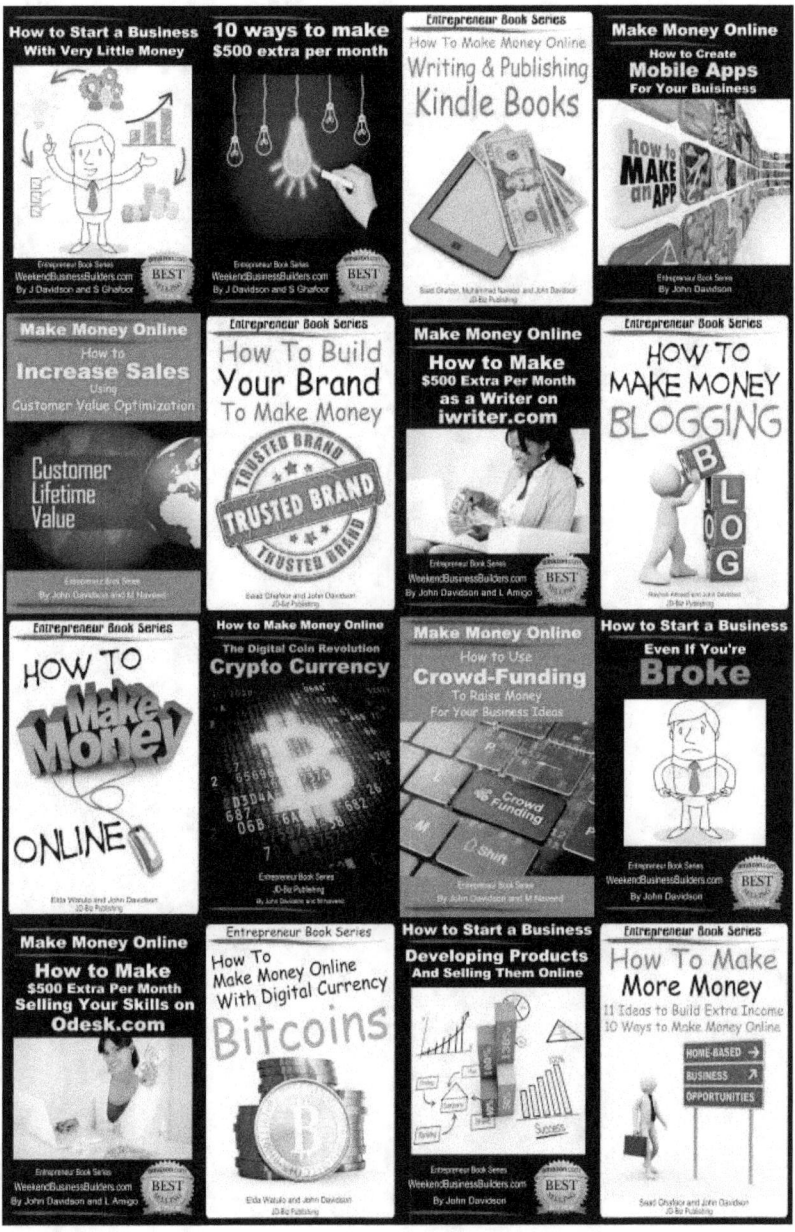

Our books are available at

1. Amazon.com

2. Barnes and Noble

3. Itunes

4. Kobo

5. Smashwords

6. Google Play Books

Download Free Books!

http://MendonCottageBooks.com

Publisher

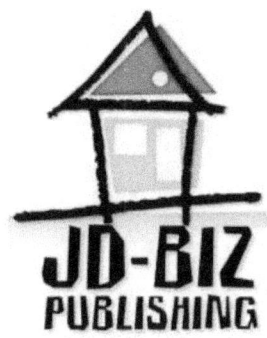

JD-Biz Corp

P O Box 374

Mendon, Utah 84325

http://www.jd-biz.com/

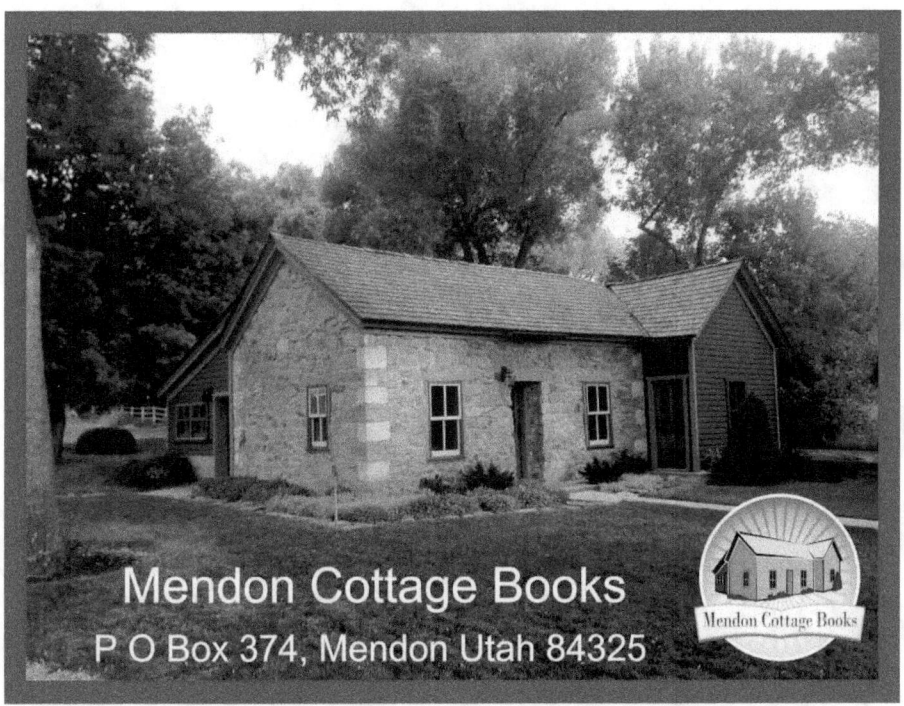

Mendon Cottage Books

P O Box 374, Mendon Utah 84325

www.ingramcontent.com/pod-product-compliance
Lightning Source LLC
Chambersburg PA
CBHW071136280526
45787CB00003B/1305